COMPLETE GUIDE TO UNDERSTANDING GALLBLADDER REMOVAL [CHOLECYSTECTOMY]

A Detailed Guide To Surgery, Postoperative Recovery, Diet, Complications, And Long-Term Health Strategies

KLEIN HOYLE

Disclaimer

The content in this book is based on the author's expertise and comprehension of the topic. The author has no affiliation or link with any corporation, business, or person. This book is meant to give general information and educational material only, and it should not be interpreted as professional medical advice. Always seek the advice of a skilled healthcare expert if you have any queries about medical issues or treatments. The author and publisher expressly disclaim any responsibility resulting directly or indirectly from the use or use of the information included in this book.

Table of Contents

ABOUT THIS BOOK

The "Complete Guide to Understanding Gallbladder Removal [Cholecystectomy]" is a beacon of information and direction for navigating the complex terrain of gallbladder health and the surgical procedures that come with it. In essence, this book is a thorough compendium, covering every aspect of cholecystectomy, from its historical beginnings to current surgical procedures and aftercare.

The first chapter introduces readers to the world of gallbladder removal, explaining the word "cholecystectomy" and its historical significance. This part not only emphasizes the need to preserve gallbladder health, but it also serves as a road map for this book's structure, enabling a seamless voyage through the complexities of the subject matter.

Chapter 2 digs more into the architecture and functions of the gallbladder, explaining the organ's critical role in digestion and bile generation. It also defines typical gallbladder disorders and the warning signals of their beginning, giving readers the information they need to identify and handle any problems early on.

Chapter 3 is a beacon of diagnostic clarity, outlining the indications and diagnostic options for cholecystectomy. Readers learn about the hazards presented by untreated gallbladder disorders via a thorough examination of surgical needs and diagnostic techniques, stressing the significance of immediate intervention.

As readers prepare for the surgical trip ahead, Chapter 4 acts as a reliable companion, providing advice on preoperative preparations such as food changes, medication adjustments, and mental fortitude. Individuals equipped with this preparation armory may face surgery with confidence and calm.

This book's core lies in Chapter 5, which methodically unpacks the whole range of gallbladder removal treatments, from classic open operations to cutting-edge robotic-assisted approaches. By illuminating the intricacies of each method, readers may make educated judgments about their chosen surgical modality.

Chapter 6 presents a thorough roadmap of what to anticipate in the operating theater, including everything from anesthetic induction to probable intraoperative difficulties. This part acts as a beacon of confidence, demystifying the surgical process and instilling a feeling of readiness.

Chapter 7 focuses on postoperative care, guiding readers through the intricacies of recovery, including pain management measures, nutritional changes, and a gradual return to regular activities. This chapter equips readers with the knowledge they need to confidently and resolutely traverse the postoperative world.

Chapter 8 faces the prospect of possible hazards and problems front on, providing information on both surgical and postoperative issues. This part acts as a beacon of empowerment, providing readers with risk-mitigation options and encouraging a proactive attitude to postoperative care.

As the path to optimum health continues, Chapter 9 emphasizes the need for postoperative care and lifestyle alterations, including advice on wound care, dietary changes, and adopting a gallbladder-friendly lifestyle. Readers may regain their health and vigor by taking a comprehensive approach to healing.

This book concludes with Chapter 10, which focuses on the long-term repercussions of gallbladder removal and the significance of follow-up treatment. This chapter guarantees that readers are on the path to long-term health and well-being by highlighting the need for continual monitoring and lifestyle changes.

CHAPTER 1

Introduction To Gallbladder Removal

What Is A Cholecystectomy?

Cholecystectomy is a surgical treatment designed to remove the gallbladder. But why should someone get their gallbladder removed? The gallbladder is a tiny organ found under the liver whose primary purpose is to retain bile generated by the liver. Bile aids in the digestion of lipids in the small intestine.

However, the gallbladder may sometimes cause complications. One typical problem is the creation of gallstones, which are hard deposits that may impede the passage of bile or even induce inflammation of the gallbladder. These gallstones may cause significant pain, nausea, and other unpleasant symptoms. In such circumstances, a cholecystectomy may be advised to relieve symptoms and avoid additional problems.

Brief History And Significance

Cholecystectomy has a long history, dating back to the nineteenth century when surgical procedures were in their infancy. The first successful cholecystectomy was conducted in 1882 by Carl Langenbuch, a German surgeon. Back then, the surgery was significantly riskier, often resulting in complications or even death.

Cholecystectomy has become a generally safe and regular surgery as medical technology and surgical procedures have advanced over time. Today, it is one of the most routinely done procedures in the world, with millions of individuals receiving the treatment annually.

The relevance of cholecystectomy stems from its capacity to cure patients of the terrible symptoms produced by gallbladder disorders. By removing the gallbladder, doctors may efficiently remove the cause of these symptoms while also improving the patient's quality of life.

Importance Of Gallbladder Health

Maintaining healthy gallbladders is critical for overall digestive health and well-being. When the gallbladder is correctly functioning, it stores and releases bile as required to help with fat digestion. However, conditions such as gallstone development or gallbladder inflammation may cause substantial pain and difficulties.

Understanding the significance of gallbladder health allows people to make efforts to avoid gallbladder disorders and preserve good digestive function. This includes following a nutritious diet high in fiber and low in saturated fats, keeping hydrated, and maintaining a healthy weight.

Regular exercise and avoiding excessive alcohol use may also help lower your chances of gallbladder problems. However, in rare circumstances, despite these precautions, surgery may still be required to treat underlying issues and relieve symptoms.

Overview Of This book's Structure

In this book, we will go further into the subject of gallbladder removal, offering a thorough guide to cholecystectomy. We will look at why someone may need to have this process, the many kinds of cholecystectomy, what to anticipate before, during, and after surgery, and advice for a smooth recovery.

In addition, we will address the dangers and implications of cholecystectomy, as well as alternate therapy options for gallbladder disorders. Whether you are considering a cholecystectomy or just want to learn more about this frequent surgical operation, this book will equip you with the knowledge you need to make educated choices about your health.

CHAPTER 2

Understanding The Gallbladder's Functions

Anatomy Of Gallbladder

The gallbladder is a tiny, pear-shaped organ found in the upper right belly, directly under the liver. Its primary purpose is to store and concentrate bile, a digestive fluid produced by the liver. The small intestine requires bile to break down lipids. The gallbladder collects bile from the liver via a system of ducts and then discharges it into the small intestine as required.

The gallbladder is made up of three primary parts: the fundus, body, and neck. The fundus is the rounded bottom region, while the body is the primary area that stores bile. The neck is a short channel that links the gallbladder with bile ducts.

Role In Digestion And Bile Production

The gallbladder performs an important function in digestion by storing and concentrating bile. When we eat fatty meals, the gallbladder contracts, and bile is released into the small intestine via the bile ducts. Bile helps to emulsify lipids, reducing them to tiny droplets that enzymes can digest more readily.

Bile aids fat digestion as well as the absorption of fat-soluble vitamins A, D, E, and K. This mechanism is essential for total nutrition absorption and maintaining healthy health.

Common Gallbladder Conditions

Several disorders may affect the gallbladder, causing symptoms and consequences. One of the most prevalent problems is gallstones, which are hardened deposits of bile that may develop in the gallbladder. Gallstones may vary in size and quantity, causing discomfort, nausea, and other digestive issues.

Other gallbladder-related illnesses include cholecystitis, which is inflammation of the gallbladder caused by gallstones, and biliary dyskinesia, a disorder characterized by irregular gallbladder contractions.

Symptoms Of Gallbladder Issues

Symptoms of gallbladder disorders vary depending on the exact ailment but often include:

1. Abdominal pain: Typically occurs in the upper right portion of the abdomen and may be acute or cramp-like.

2. Nausea and vomiting: Especially after consuming fatty meals.

3. Indigestion: Difficulty digesting fatty meals, which causes bloating and discomfort.

4. Jaundice is the yellowing of the skin and eyes caused by bile duct blockage.

5. Fever and chills are common signs of acute cholecystitis, an inflammation of the gallbladder.

If you encounter any of these symptoms, you should get medical assistance right once, since untreated gallbladder issues may lead to consequences including infection, pancreatitis, or even a burst gallbladder.

Understanding the architecture and function of the gallbladder, as well as detecting indicators of possible problems, is critical for maintaining digestive health and obtaining prompt medical attention when needed.

CHAPTER 3

Indications And Diagnosis Of Cholecystectomy

When Surgery Is Essential

Cholecystectomy, or surgical removal of the gallbladder, is indicated when gallbladder problems continue and have a major influence on a person's health and quality of life. Surgery is usually advised for those who have recurring gallstones, significant gallbladder inflammation (cholecystitis), or complications such as pancreatitis or gallbladder malignancy.

One of the key causes of surgery is the existence of gallstones, which cause pain and suffering. If these stones clog the bile ducts, they might cause serious consequences such as infection or inflammation. In such circumstances, removing the gallbladder is often the most efficient way to avoid additional issues and relieve discomfort.

Diagnostic Procedures

Before proposing cholecystectomy, healthcare experts use a variety of diagnostic techniques to diagnose gallbladder disorders and assess the need for surgery.

1. Ultrasound: This non-invasive imaging technique is widely used to examine the gallbladder and find gallstones. Ultrasound identifies the size, shape, and condition of the gallbladder, which is useful for diagnosis and therapy planning.

2. Blood tests may be used to evaluate liver function and identify evidence of inflammation or infection. Elevated levels of specific enzymes may suggest gallbladder abnormalities, allowing doctors to make an educated judgment about whether surgery is necessary.

3. CT scan or MRI: In certain circumstances, further imaging tests such as computed tomography (CT) scans or magnetic resonance imaging (MRI) may be used to get detailed pictures of the gallbladder and surrounding organs. These tests may help uncover issues including gallbladder inflammation or bile duct obstructions.

Identifying Gallbladder Diseases

Cholecystectomy is often indicated for a variety of gallbladder illnesses that have a serious impact on a person's health and well-being. Some of the frequent problems that may justify surgical removal of the gallbladder are:

1. Gallstones are hardened deposits of digestive fluid that may accumulate in the gallbladder. Gallstones may induce stomach discomfort, nausea, vomiting, and jaundice. If left untreated, gallstones may cause cholecystitis, pancreatitis, and bile duct blockage.

2. Cholecystitis is inflammation of the gallbladder caused by gallstones that clog the bile ducts. If not addressed, cholecystitis may cause severe stomach discomfort, fever, and even death. Surgery is often required to remove an inflamed gallbladder and avoid future occurrences.

3. Gallbladder cancer: Although uncommon, gallbladder cancer may need surgical removal of the gallbladder, particularly if found early enough. Surgery may be coupled with other therapies, such as chemotherapy or radiation therapy, to enhance results.

Risks Of Not Treating Gallbladder Problems

Leaving gallbladder disorders untreated may have major repercussions, including complications that damage both health and quality of life. Untreated gallbladder problems may provide the following risks:

1. **Pain and discomfort:** Gallstones and inflammation may cause chronic stomach pain, nausea, and vomiting, limiting daily activities and quality of life.

2. **Complications:** Untreated gallbladder problems may result in cholecystitis, pancreatitis, bile duct blockage, or even gallbladder rupture. These consequences may need immediate medical attention and might be fatal if not treated quickly.

3. Prolonged exposure to gallbladder troubles may lead to the development of chronic health concerns such as liver damage, digestive disorders, and an increased chance of gallbladder cancer.

4. **Reduced quality of life:** The persistent symptoms and consequences of untreated gallbladder disease may hurt physical health, emotional well-being, and overall quality of life. Surgical removal of the gallbladder is often required to relieve symptoms, avoid complications, and enhance long-term results.

Understanding the grounds for cholecystectomy and the hazards of leaving gallbladder problems untreated is critical for making educated treatment choices and maintaining optimum health and well-being. If you have symptoms that imply a gallbladder condition, you should see a doctor for an accurate diagnosis and treatment. Early detection and timely treatment may help avoid complications and improve overall results for people with gallbladder problems.

CHAPTER 4

Preparing For Gallbladder Surgery

Preoperative Assessments And Evaluations

Before gallbladder surgery, also known as cholecystectomy, many preoperative exams and evaluations are performed to verify that the patient is physically ready for the treatment and to detect any possible risks or problems.

One of the key examinations is a detailed medical history review, which documents the patient's prior medical illnesses, surgeries, allergies, and prescriptions. This allows the medical staff to better understand the patient's general health and any issues that may impact the operation or anesthesia.

Physical exams are also used to determine the patient's current health state. This may involve vital sign readings such as blood pressure, heart rate, and temperature, as well as a comprehensive abdominal examination to look for symptoms of inflammation or pain that might signal gallbladder issues.

Furthermore, laboratory tests such as blood tests, urine analysis, and imaging studies such as ultrasound or CT scans may be ordered to assess the condition of the gallbladder and surrounding organs, as well as the patient's overall health, and identify any underlying medical issues that must be addressed before surgery.

These preoperative exams and evaluations are critical for ensuring that the patient is well-prepared for gallbladder surgery and that any possible risks or problems are detected and addressed appropriately.

Dietary And Lifestyle Changes Before Surgery

Making dietary and lifestyle adjustments before gallbladder surgery may improve the procedure's success and speed up the healing period. One of the most significant dietary modifications is to avoid fatty and greasy meals, which may worsen gallbladder symptoms and raise the risk of problems before and after surgery.

Instead, patients are recommended to eat a low-fat diet in the days before surgery. This usually contains lean meats like chicken, fish, and tofu, as well as a variety of fruits, vegetables, and complete grains. Avoiding fried meals, processed foods, and high-fat dairy items may help lessen the gallbladder's burden and lower the chance of gallstone issues.

In addition to dietary adjustments, patients should maintain a healthy lifestyle before gallbladder surgery. This includes sticking to a regular exercise schedule, being hydrated, and avoiding smoking and excessive alcohol intake. These lifestyle changes may help improve general health and fitness, resulting in an easier recovery after surgery.

Patients should also follow their healthcare provider's particular recommendations for fasting before surgery and taking any prescribed medicines. By following these dietary and lifestyle suggestions, patients may help ensure the success of their gallbladder surgery while also promoting optimum healing and recovery.

Medications And Supplements To Avoid

Before having gallbladder surgery, patients should be informed of which drugs and supplements to avoid in the days preceding the operation. Certain drugs and supplements might raise the risk of bleeding or other issues after surgery, so it's critical to follow your doctor's instructions carefully.

Nonsteroidal anti-inflammatory medicines (NSAIDs) like ibuprofen and aspirin should be avoided in the days before gallbladder surgery because they may interfere with blood coagulation and raise the risk of severe bleeding during the operation. Instead, patients may be advised to use acetaminophen for pain relief, since it has a lower influence on blood clotting.

Additionally, herbal supplements and alternative therapies should be avoided before surgery since they may include substances that interfere with the anesthetic or other prescriptions used during the operation. It is important to notify your healthcare practitioner about any supplements or herbal therapies you are currently taking so that they can advise you on which to quit before surgery.

In rare situations, patients may need to temporarily discontinue prescription drugs before gallbladder surgery, especially if they are blood thinners or have other possible complications with anesthesia. Your healthcare practitioner will offer particular advice depending on your medical history and current medicines.

Patients who avoid certain drugs and supplements before gallbladder surgery may help reduce the risk of problems and guarantee a safe and successful treatment.

Mental And Emotional Preparation

Preparing for gallbladder surgery requires not only physical but also mental and emotional preparation. Surgery may be a frightening experience for many individuals, so it's important to make efforts to lessen worry and tension in the run-up to the surgery.

One method to psychologically prepare for gallbladder surgery is to learn about the process and what to anticipate before, during, and after it. This may assist in relieving anxieties and doubts by offering a clear picture of the procedure and what is involved.

Talking with your healthcare professional about any worries or questions you may have may also help to reduce anxiety and give confidence. Your healthcare team is there to assist you during the surgical procedure and may provide assistance and advice to help you feel more confident and prepared.

Deep breathing, meditation, and yoga are all relaxation practices that may help quiet the mind and decrease tension before surgery. These approaches may be especially useful in the days preceding the surgery, when anxiety may be at its highest.

It is also critical to have a solid support structure in place before gallbladder surgery. This might include family members, friends, or support groups that can provide emotional support and encouragement during the medical procedure and recuperation time.

CHAPTER 5

Gallbladder Removal Procedures

Laparoscopic Cholecystectomy

Laparoscopic cholecystectomy is a minimally invasive surgical technique that removes the gallbladder. It is the most popular approach for gallbladder removal nowadays owing to its various benefits over conventional open surgery. In this surgery, the surgeon creates small incisions in the belly and inserts a tiny camera known as a laparoscope, as well as specialized surgical equipment. The camera gives a magnified picture of the interior of the abdomen, enabling the surgeon to observe and maneuver the operating region precisely.

One of the primary advantages of laparoscopic cholecystectomy is that it requires less recovery time than open surgery.

Because the incisions are smaller and fewer, patients usually endure less discomfort and scarring. Furthermore, since the technique is less invasive, problems like infection and bleeding are reduced.

During the operation, the surgeon fills the belly with carbon dioxide gas to make room for the surgery. The gallbladder is then delicately removed from the liver and surrounding organs using laparoscopic devices. Once the gallbladder has been released, it is removed via one of the tiny incisions. In rare circumstances, a drainage tube may be temporarily inserted near the surgical site to assist remove excess fluid.

Following gallbladder removal, the wounds are closed with sutures or surgical adhesive, and the patient is typically allowed to go home the same day or after a brief hospital stay. Most patients may return to their usual activities within a week or two, although vigorous activity and heavy lifting should be avoided for a few weeks to allow for adequate healing.

Open Cholecystectomy

Open cholecystectomy is a classic surgical procedure for gallbladder removal that requires a bigger incision in the abdomen. While it is less prevalent nowadays because of the extensive use of laparoscopic procedures, it may still be required in certain circumstances when laparoscopic surgery is neither practical nor safe.

An open cholecystectomy involves the surgeon making a single big incision in the upper belly, which is often several inches long. This incision gives the surgeon immediate access to the gallbladder and its surrounding tissues, enabling him to safely remove it.

Although open cholecystectomy has a wider incision and may cause more discomfort and scarring than laparoscopic surgery, it remains a very successful therapy for gallbladder illness. It may be preferable in situations when the patient has significant gallbladder inflammation or scarring, or if there are problems such as gallstones stuck in the bile ducts.

Following gallbladder removal, the incision is closed with sutures or staples, and the patient is usually observed in the hospital for a few days to ensure good healing. The recovery period for open cholecystectomy is greater than for laparoscopic surgery, with most patients requiring several weeks to completely recover and resume regular activities.

Robotic Assisted Cholecystectomy

Robotic-assisted cholecystectomy is a relatively new technique for gallbladder removal that combines the advantages of laparoscopic surgery with the accuracy and dexterity of robotic technology. In this operation, the surgeon sits at a console and directs robotic arms carrying surgical equipment, while a camera offers a three-dimensional picture of the operative site.

One of the primary benefits of robotic-assisted cholecystectomy is increased accuracy and control, allowing for more accurate tissue motions and manipulation than conventional laparoscopic surgery. This may be especially useful when the gallbladder is difficult to reach if there are intricate anatomical variances.

Another benefit of robotic surgery is its ergonomic design, which may help doctors avoid tiredness and hand tremors during protracted operations. This may result in improved patient outcomes and reduced operating times.

Similar to laparoscopic cholecystectomy, robotic-assisted cholecystectomy is less invasive, with smaller incisions and quicker recovery periods than open surgery. However, it may not be appropriate for all individuals, especially those with certain medical issues or anatomical constraints.

Nonsurgical Alternatives

Non-surgical treatment options for gallbladder illness include medicines and lithotripsy. Medications may be provided to dissolve gallstones or to treat symptoms like pain and inflammation. However, these drugs are often only helpful for certain kinds of gallstones and may take many months to act.

Lithotripsy is a non-surgical therapy that employs shock waves to break down gallstones into smaller fragments that may subsequently move naturally via the digestive system. This technique is often reserved for individuals who are not good candidates for surgery or who choose to forgo surgery entirely.

While non-surgical treatments may provide immediate relief from symptoms, they are not considered a long-term cure for gallbladder illness. In most situations, surgical removal of the gallbladder is indicated to avoid future issues such as gallstone infections or bile duct obstructions.

CHAPTER 6

The Surgery Procedure: What To Expect

Anesthesia And Operation Room Procedures

Before gallbladder removal surgery, you will be given an anesthetic to keep you comfortable and pain-free during the process. There are several forms of anesthetic, and your medical team will choose the best one depending on your health status and the intricacy of the operation.

Once in the operating room, the anesthesiologist will carefully monitor your vital signs, such as heart rate, blood pressure, and oxygen levels, to guarantee your safety during the process. They will then deliver the anesthetic, which might be general anesthesia (where you are fully asleep) or regional anesthesia (when just a portion of your body is numb).

After the anesthetic has taken effect, the surgical team will place you on the operating table and sterilize the surgical site to limit the risk of infection. They will wrap your body with sterile drapes, leaving just the operation location exposed.

Steps Of The Surgical Procedure

The surgical treatment for gallbladder removal, known as cholecystectomy, may be done using a variety of procedures, including laparoscopic and open surgery. The particular approach used is determined by criteria such as the patient's medical history, the occurrence of problems, and the surgeon's experience.

A laparoscopic cholecystectomy involves the surgeon making many tiny incisions in the belly and inserting a laparoscope—a thin, flexible tube with a camera and light attached—through one of the incisions. This permits the surgical team to see the gallbladder and its surrounding structures on a monitor.

The surgeon delicately removes the gallbladder from the liver and bile ducts using specialist equipment put via the other incisions. Once totally disengaged, the gallbladder is removed via one of the incisions. The incisions are subsequently sealed with sutures or surgical adhesive.

Open cholecystectomy involves the surgeon making a single major incision in the belly to get direct access to the gallbladder. This procedure may be required if the gallbladder is inflamed, infected, or there are problems.

Duration Of Surgery

The time of gallbladder removal surgery varies based on the patient's anatomy, the existence of comorbidities, and the surgical method used. On average, a laparoscopic cholecystectomy takes 60 to 90 minutes to perform, but an open cholecystectomy might take up to 120 minutes.

It is important to note that the time of the operation is just one component of the whole procedure. Preoperative preparations, such as medical examinations and anesthetic administration, will take place before surgery, and you will be carefully watched throughout the postoperative period to ensure adequate recovery.

Potential Intraoperative Complications

Although gallbladder removal surgery is typically safe, it does include certain risks. Bleeding, harm to nearby organs such as the bile duct or intestine, and anesthesia-related adverse responses are all possible intraoperative problems.

To reduce the risk of problems, your surgical team will take several measures, including thorough patient evaluation, adherence to surgical guidelines, and constant monitoring throughout the treatment.

CHAPTER 7

Recovery Following Gallbladder Removal

Hospital Stay Duration

Your hospital stay after gallbladder removal surgery may vary based on various variables, including the kind of surgery conducted, your general health, and any issues that may emerge during or after the treatment. Laparoscopic cholecystectomy, the most frequent approach, often needs a shorter hospital stay than open surgery.

Patients who undergo simple laparoscopic cholecystectomy generally spend 1 to 2 days in the hospital. During this time, medical personnel will check your vital signs, prescribe pain medication as required, and ensure that you are healing well following surgery. If there are no issues and you can eat, drink, and walk about comfortably, you may be released sooner.

If an open cholecystectomy is done, or if difficulties arise during surgery, such as heavy bleeding or trouble removing the gallbladder, your hospital stay may be extended, ranging from 2 to 5 days or more. Your medical team will continuously monitor your health and offer any required treatment until you are stable enough to be released.

Pain Management Strategies

Pain management is an important part of the recovery process following gallbladder removal surgery to maintain your comfort and promote healing. It is common and anticipated to feel discomfort or pain in the belly, shoulder, or back immediately after surgery. Your doctor will prescribe pain medication to ease these symptoms.

To treat mild to moderate pain, over-the-counter or prescription pain medications such as acetaminophen (Tylenol) or nonsteroidal anti-inflammatory medicines (NSAIDs) like ibuprofen are usually prescribed. For more severe pain, your doctor may prescribe stronger drugs such as opioids, although they are typically used for a limited period owing to the risk of addiction and other adverse effects.

In addition to medicine, alternative pain management treatments may include applying cold packs to the surgical site, using heating pads to relax muscles, and practicing relaxation techniques like deep breathing exercises or guided imagery to decrease tension and enhance healing.

Dietary Guidelines For Recovery

A good diet is essential for a successful recovery after gallbladder removal surgery. While your body adapts to the loss of the gallbladder, it is important to follow dietary advice to avoid digestive pain and encourage recovery.

Immediately after surgery, your healthcare professional may prescribe a clear liquid diet consisting of broth, gelatin, clear juices, and plain water to enable your digestive system to rest and gradually reintroduce foods. As you grow, you may transition to a completely liquid diet, which includes yogurt, pudding, and blended soups.

Once you can handle liquids well, you may gradually switch to a soft, low-fat diet rich in readily digested foods like lean protein, cooked vegetables, fruits, whole grains, and healthy fats like olive oil. It is essential to avoid fatty, greasy, fried, and spicy meals since they might aggravate digestive problems like diarrhea or indigestion, particularly in the absence of the gallbladder.

As your body heals, you may gradually reintroduce normal foods into your diet, but be sure to listen to your body and avoid anything that causes pain or stomach distress. Consulting with a licensed dietitian may also help you create a tailored food plan that fulfills your nutritional requirements and promotes your recovery.

Resuming Normal Activities

Recovery following gallbladder removal surgery is gradually returning to regular activities while giving your body time to recuperate. During the first recovery phase, it's critical to obtain enough rest and avoid intense activity that might strain your abdominal muscles or impede healing.

Your healthcare practitioner will provide you precise guidelines on when you may progressively increase your activity level depending on your unique healing status. Light exercises like walking or moderate stretching may usually be resumed a few days following surgery to improve circulation and avoid blood clots.

Depending on how you feel, as you rebuild strength and stamina, you may gradually add more moderate tasks such as housework, mild exercise, and returning to work. It's important to listen to your body and pace yourself while avoiding activities that cause pain or discomfort.

While it is common to feel fatigued and limited in the weeks after surgery, most individuals may gradually resume their usual activities within 4 to 6 weeks. However, if you have chronic discomfort, fever, severe exhaustion, or other symptoms, you should see your healthcare professional for additional examination and assistance.

CHAPTER 8
Possible Risks And Complications

Surgical Complications

Surgical complications are dangers that might occur during or after a cholecystectomy operation. Complications may include bleeding, infection, or organ damage. During the procedure, the surgeon delicately dissects the tissues around the gallbladder to remove it without causing damage to the surrounding structures. However, even with safeguards, there is still a danger of bleeding from blood vessels severed during the process.

Infection is another worry after surgery. Despite the use of sterile methods and medicines, there is a slight chance of developing an infection at the surgical site or in the abdomen. This danger is generally decreased by adequate wound care and medicines as indicated by the surgeon.

Furthermore, injury to neighboring organs such as the liver or bile ducts might occur during surgery, resulting in further issues that may need multiple treatments to resolve.

Postoperative Complications

Postoperative problems arise after the procedure is done. A frequent postoperative consequence of cholecystectomy is bile duct damage. The bile ducts are fragile structures that transport bile from the liver to the small intestine. If these ducts are unintentionally cut or damaged during surgery, bile may seep into the abdominal cavity, causing discomfort, infection, and other significant problems.

Bile leakage is another postoperative problem that may arise after cholecystectomy. This may occur if the bile ducts are not correctly sealed or if they rip during surgery. If bile leakage is not addressed immediately, it might cause infection and other issues. Patients who have symptoms such as stomach discomfort, fever, or jaundice after surgery should seek medical assistance right once to rule out bile leakage and other problems.

Long-Term Risks

While cholecystectomy is widely regarded as safe and successful for treating gallbladder disorders, there are some long-term hazards to consider. One such danger is the onset of stomach problems. Without a gallbladder, the body may have difficulties digesting certain meals, especially fatty or oily ones. This may cause symptoms including diarrhea, bloating, and gas.

Another long-term danger is the development of new gallstones. Even after the gallbladder has been removed, gallstones may still develop in the bile ducts or liver. These stones may cause discomfort and other difficulties if they become trapped in the ducts or obstruct the passage of bile. Doctors may prescribe dietary adjustments or drugs to assist control of bile production and composition to lessen the chance of developing new gallstones.

Strategies For Risk Reduction

Numerous measures may be used to lessen the risk of problems during and after cholecystectomy. One crucial method is to choose an experienced surgeon who has conducted several cholecystectomy operations and is acquainted with the architecture of the gallbladder and its surrounding components. Furthermore, patients may lower their risk of problems according to their surgeon's preoperative instructions, which may include fasting before surgery and discontinuing certain drugs that raise the risk of bleeding.

Advanced surgical procedures, such as laparoscopy, may assist limit tissue damage while also lowering the risk of bleeding and infection. Following surgery, patients should carefully follow their surgeon's postoperative recommendations, which include taking prescribed medicines, keeping the surgical site clean and dry, and refraining from heavy activities until completely healed. Patients who follow these techniques may reduce their risk of complications and obtain a satisfactory result after cholecystectomy.

CHAPTER 9

Post-Operative Care And Lifestyle Changes

Wound Care And Monitoring

Following a cholecystectomy, adequate wound care is essential for a successful recovery. Your healthcare practitioner will most likely offer specific advice on how to care for your incision areas. Generally, it entails keeping the wounds clean and dry. You may be recommended to gently wash the area with mild soap and water before patting it dry with a clean towel.

Monitor your incision sites for symptoms of infection, such as increased redness, edema, temperature, or pus leakage. If you have any of these symptoms or develop a fever, you should contact your healthcare professional immediately. They may need to examine the wound and give antibiotics if required.

It is typical to feel some discomfort or minor pain around the incision sites as they heal. Your healthcare professional may suggest over-the-counter pain medications or prescription medicine to assist you manage any pain or discomfort.

Gradual Reintroduction Of Foods

After a cholecystectomy, you may need to gradually reintroduce foods into your diet to let your body acclimate to the changes. Your healthcare physician or a qualified dietitian may advise you on which foods to start with and how to advance to a more diverse diet.

Initially, you may be encouraged to consume bland, low-fat meals that are simple to digest, such as broth-based soups, plain rice, boiled potatoes, and lean meats such as chicken or fish. As your body adjusts to these meals, you may gradually reintroduce additional foods such as fruits, vegetables, whole grains, and dairy products.

It's important to listen to your body and observe how various meals make you feel. You may notice that some meals cause digestive problems like bloating, gas, or diarrhea. If this happens, you may need to avoid or restrict certain items in your diet.

Importance Of Hydration And Exercise

Staying hydrated is critical for the healing process and general health after a cholecystectomy. Drinking enough water helps to avoid dehydration, which may exacerbate constipation and other digestive disorders that may arise after surgery.

Your healthcare physician may advise you to gradually increase your activity level while you recuperate from surgery. Light physical activity, like as walking or light stretching exercises, may help avoid issues like blood clots and speed up recovery.

It is critical to adhere to your healthcare provider's advice for physical activity and avoid activities that may strain or put pressure on your abdominal muscles until you have completely healed. Remember to listen to your body and discontinue any activity that produces pain or discomfort.

Adopting A Gallbladder-Friendly Diet

Following a cholecystectomy, eating a gallbladder-friendly diet may help reduce digestive problems and improve overall health. This usually entails eating a well-balanced diet that is low in fat and rich in fiber.

Fiber-rich foods, such as fruits, vegetables, whole grains, and legumes, may help encourage regular bowel movements and reduce constipation following gallbladder removal. It is important to consume healthy fats such as avocados, nuts, seeds, and fatty fish while avoiding fried and greasy meals, which may worsen digestive problems.

In addition to dietary choices, it's crucial to consider portion sizes and meal scheduling. Eating smaller, more frequent meals throughout the day may assist in avoiding overloading your digestive system and relieving pain.

You may encourage a smooth recovery and enhance digestive health after gallbladder removal by making incremental adjustments to your food and lifestyle, as well as following your healthcare provider's postoperative care recommendations.

CHAPTER 10

Long-Term Effects And Follow-Up Care

Impact On Digestion And Bile Regulation

Following a cholecystectomy, it's normal to question how the removal of your gallbladder may affect your digestion and bile flow. Let us break it down.

Your gallbladder is essential to the digestive process because it stores and concentrates bile, a fluid generated by the liver that aids in fat digestion. Even without a gallbladder, your liver still produces bile, which passes straight into your small intestine. This means that, although you may notice some changes in how your body processes fats, such as occasional diarrhea or more frequent bowel motions, most individuals adjust well to the loss of their gallbladder over time.

In the lack of a gallbladder, bile is discharged into the small intestine in a steady trickle rather than in concentrated bursts after a meal. Some individuals may need to modify their diet to meet this shift. For example, you may benefit from eating smaller, more often meals rather than big, greasy meals, which might overload your digestive system.

Some people may also have bile reflux, which occurs when bile rushes backward into the stomach rather than into the small intestine. This might sometimes result in symptoms like heartburn or stomach pain. If you have these symptoms regularly, your doctor may suggest drugs or dietary changes to help you manage them.

Overall, although the lack of a gallbladder may require some early adaptations in digestion and bile management, most patients find that they can live normal, healthy lives with little disturbance.

Monitoring For Complications

Following a cholecystectomy, it is critical to watch for any possible problems that may occur. Here's what you should know.

One possible consequence is bile duct damage, which may occur during the procedure. This might result in complications like bile leakage or obstruction, which may need extra operations to resolve. Bile duct damage symptoms may include stomach discomfort, fever, jaundice (yellowing of the skin or eyes), nausea, and vomiting. If you suffer any of these symptoms after your operation, you should immediately contact your healthcare practitioner.

Another potential consequence is the production of gallstones in the bile ducts, often known as retained or recurring stones. While gallbladder removal often inhibits the production of new gallstones, old stones may still get trapped in the bile ducts. This might result in symptoms including stomach discomfort, jaundice, or pancreatitis. If you encounter any of these symptoms, get medical care right once.

In addition to monitoring for surgery-related complications, keep an eye out for any indicators of digestive difficulties or other concerns that may occur after your cholecystectomy. If you have persistent symptoms such as stomach discomfort, diarrhea, or problems digesting particular meals, contact your healthcare professional for advice.

Follow-Up Consultations And Testing

Following a cholecystectomy, you will most likely need to schedule follow-up meetings with your healthcare practitioner to verify that you are recovering appropriately and to monitor for any possible issues. Here's what to anticipate.

Your initial follow-up visit will usually occur within a few weeks following your surgery. During this session, your healthcare practitioner will examine your incision sites, look for signs of infection or other problems, and talk about any symptoms or concerns you have. They may also request blood tests or imaging investigations to assess your liver's function and rule out any leftover gallstones or other abnormalities.

In the months and years after your surgery, you may need to visit your doctor regularly for normal check-ups. These consultations are critical for monitoring your general health and ensuring that you do not develop any long-term issues from your cholecystectomy.

In addition to follow-up meetings with your doctor, you may need to have frequent imaging tests, such as ultrasounds or MRI scans, to check the condition of your liver and bile ducts. These tests may discover possible abnormalities early on, allowing for timely action if necessary.

Lifestyle Changes For Good Health

Following a cholecystectomy, implementing some lifestyle changes might help you maintain your overall health and wellness. Here are some pointers to consider.

First and foremost, it's important to eat a healthy, balanced diet. While you may not need to adhere to a strict low-fat diet after your surgery, you may discover that certain foods are easier to digest than others. Experiment with various meals to determine what works best for you, and be sure to include lots of fruits, vegetables, healthy grains, and lean meats in your diet.

In addition to consuming a balanced diet, frequent exercise is essential for maintaining good health after a cholecystectomy. On most days of the week, aim to do at least 30 minutes of moderate aerobic activity, such as walking, swimming, or cycling. Exercise not only promotes a healthy weight and cardiovascular health, but it may also assist with digestion and general well-being.

Finally, listen to your body and be aware of any symptoms or changes in your health that may occur after your operation. If you are experiencing chronic stomach discomfort, digestive issues, or other concerns, do not hesitate to contact your healthcare professional for advice and assistance. Following a cholecystectomy, you may live a full and active life by making proactive efforts to maintain your health and well-being.

Conclusion

The end of a thorough guide to understanding gallbladder removal, or cholecystectomy, includes numerous crucial points that emphasize the procedure's importance and repercussions for patients.

To begin, cholecystectomy is a frequent surgical treatment used to treat the symptoms and problems of gallbladder disease, such as gallstones. Patients who have their gallbladder removed may have relief from discomfort, digestive problems, and possible consequences such as infections or inflammation caused by gallstones.

Second, although cholecystectomy is typically deemed safe and successful, patients must be fully educated about the treatment, including its risks and benefits. Understanding the reasons for having a cholecystectomy, the various methods of surgery (laparoscopic vs. open), and the healing period may help patients make educated choices in partnership with their doctors.

Furthermore, the advice highlights the need for post-operative care and lifestyle changes after a cholecystectomy. Patients are often encouraged to eat a balanced, low-fat diet to avoid intestinal pain and to gradually resume physical activity as they heal. Furthermore, some individuals may suffer changes in bowel habits or dietary tolerances after gallbladder surgery, necessitating continued discussion with healthcare experts to address any issues or difficulties.

Furthermore, the guide's conclusion emphasizes the need to schedule frequent follow-up meetings with healthcare specialists to evaluate healing progress and handle any remaining symptoms or consequences. While most patients see a considerable improvement in their quality of life after cholecystectomy, rare complications such as bile duct damage or post-cholecystectomy syndrome may need further medical intervention.

Finally, the conclusion highlights the significance of patient education and empowerment in navigating the journey before, during, and after cholecystectomy. Patients may improve their results and reduce the risk of problems by understanding the purpose of the surgery, actively engaging in treatment choices, and following post-operative protocols.

In conclusion, the complete guide to understanding gallbladder removal emphasizes the transformative impact of cholecystectomy on patients' lives, the importance of informed decision-making and post-operative care, and the role of ongoing communication between patients and healthcare providers in achieving optimal outcomes.

THE END